CANNABINOID ABUSE AND MISUSE:

ITS CONNECTED IMPACT ON HEALTH AND WELL-BEING. .

First Published, 2023

Noogul Digital Publishing

Edited by:

Ishaku Usman Gadzama PhD

Senior Lecturer,

Department of Sociology, Faculty of Social Sciences,

Ahmadu Bello University, Zaria, Kaduna State

Nigeria

Email: iugadzama@gmail.com

Dr. Okoosi Sunday Adegoke

Human Physiologist

Ahmadu Bello University Teaching Hospital, Zaria.

Kaduna State, Nigeria

Email: sundayokoosi@yahoo.com

Preface

Cannabinoid Abuse and Misuse: Its Connected Impact on Health and Well-Being is an abridged *version of Substance Abuse and Substance Use Disorders: A Global Pandemic among Teenagers and youths: Implications for Counselling.* This book made clear how to deal with today's substance-related problems. Abuse of substances and drugs, along with the accompanying physical, social, and mental diseases, has emerged as a global issue. The "Innovative Substances" disclosed in this book have given the issues with drugs, particularly socio-demographic borders, new dimensions.

For the benefit of his broad target audience's reading and understanding, the author has imaginatively categorized cannabinoids in this book using the most comprehensible typology. The book dedicates each Section and Unit to a class, offering a brief history of the class, its Chemical Structures, forms, kinds, and pathogenetic sequences, as well as how to identify symptoms and treat misuse and addiction as well as diseases that are associated to them.

The book should appeal to readers because of its simple layout. The book will be of great use to professionals in the social sciences, education, health, and other helping professions..

Additionally, every family should read and maintain a copy.

Emmanuel Ejembi Anyebe PhD, JP.

Associate Professor,

Mental Health Unit, Department of Nursing Sciences,

Faculty of Clinical Sciences,

College of Health Sciences, University of Ilorin

Ilorin 240001,Nigeria.

Mobile: +2348036422771

Email: ejembianyebe@gmail.com; anyebe.ee@unilorin.edu.ng

TABLE OF CONTENTS

SECTION ONE

DRUG MISUSE, DRUG ABUSE AND ADDICTION

Introduction

Addiction, drug abuse, and misuse are all major public health issues. Many individuals frequently use these phrases interchangeably since they all relate to the use of illicit drugs as well as the improper use of legal substances (such as cigarettes, alcohol, and prescription medications). But each issue's interventions differ substantially from one another. The importance of accurately diagnosing a person's drug use is due to this. Medication on prescription has a lot of positive impacts. They can make us live longer, healthier lives when used properly under medical care. However, these same drugs have the capacity to have fatal results and serious adverse effects, particularly when overused or abused. Prescription drugs should only be taken by the individual for whom they are designed and exactly as directed due to this risk of damage.

Drug Misuse

Prescription medications are commonly related with drug misuse. Prescription medications are intended to be taken exactly as prescribed by doctors. This is because these medications might have negative side effects if the instructions are not followed.

Drug Misuse occurs when these drugs are used for purposes that are not in accordance with legal or medical norms.

- Taking the wrong dose
- Taking the medication at the wrong time
- Forgetting to take a dose
- Stopping the usage of a drug too soon
- Taking a medicine for reasons other than those indicated
- Taking a drug that was not prescribed to you

The FDA (2019) defines prescription medication MISUSE as failing to follow medical directions, although the individual using the medicine is not intending to "get high." If a person is unable to fall asleep after taking a single sleeping tablet, they may take another pill an hour later, reasoning, "That will do the job." Alternatively, a person may offer his headache medicine to a buddy in agony. Those are examples of drug abuse because, according to the FDA, the individual is treating oneself but not in accordance with the recommendations of their health care professionals. Prescription medication abuse can include: taking the wrong dose; taking a dose at the wrong time; forgetting to take a dose; and discontinuing medicine too soon, according to the Institute for Safe Medication Practices.

Drug Abuse

Drug abuse occurs when any psychoactive substance, including alcohol, illegal narcotics, and prescription medications, is used improperly to get high or hurt oneself. Since drug user's exhibit profoundly changed thinking, behavior, and bodily functioning, it is also known as substance use disorder (SUD). According to the National Institute on Drug Abuse (NIDA, 2019), prescription drug abuse is the use of a medicine without a prescription, in a manner other than as directed, or for the experience or sensations it produces. For instance, drug abuse occurs when someone consumes a prescription medication in larger dosages than recommended in order to "get high" or have a pleasant or euphoric feeling.

The primary distinction between someone who misuses drugs and someone who abuses drugs is their purpose. The former consumes a medicine to cure a specific condition, whereas the latter consumes a substance to provoke specific emotions.

When a person fails to fall asleep after taking one sleeping pill and takes another one an hour later in the hopes that "it'll do the job," this is an example of drug abuse. But when someone uses sleeping drugs to regulate their moods, get a "high," or, in the worst-case circumstances, to attempt suicide, that is drug addiction.

Drug Addiction

Drug addiction, often referred to as severe SUD, is a brain illness that shows itself as the inability to stop using a substance despite the negative effects. Because they experience severe or incapacitating withdrawal symptoms when they stop using a substance, those who are addicted to drugs have a physical and/or psychological desire to use that substance.

Your brain and behavior are both impacted by the condition of addiction. Substance addiction makes it unable to resist the impulse to use the drug, regardless of how harmful it may be. The sooner you receive treatment for drug addiction, the better your chances are of avoiding some of the disease's more serious side effects.

Not simply heroin, cocaine, or other illicit narcotics are involved in drug addiction. Alcohol, nicotine, sleep aids, anti-anxiety drugs, and other legal substances can all cause addiction.

Drug misuse can take the form of addiction. The ability of the user to manage oneself is what distinguishes the two disorders. A person abusing drugs doesn't face a significant upheaval in their life since they still have control over it.

The majority, if not all, parts of a person's life are affected by an addiction, in contrast. Due to their substance use, they frequently skip job or school, put their families in financial or physical risk, experience health difficulties, encounter legal challenges, and engage in other hazardous behaviors. However, despite these, they are unable to alter their routines in order to improve their circumstances. This explains why a lot of drug addicts lose their jobs, end up homeless, or split up from their families. Some people's drug addiction even results in death.

Progression In Drug Use

An addiction does not appear out of nowhere. Instead, it is the outcome of a protracted period of continuous substance usage that gradually alters how a person perceives drugs and how their bodies react to them. This process is linear and follows the same pattern for everyone, albeit the length of each step varies widely depending on the individual, dosage, and type of drug being abused.

Because this process follows a pattern, it may be divided into stages that lead to addiction, beginning with the first use and ending with the addiction itself. While there is considerable disagreement over how many stages there are in addiction, seven is one of the most commonly used numbers to describe the process.

The natural history of drug use can be divided into five categories: ***first use, continued use, consequences, dependence and addiction, and cessation and recovery***. Some of these processes may occur multiple times for the same or other substances during the lifespan of a dependent user. The primary characteristics that impact drug use careers and the repercussions connected with it are of particular relevance since they may have significant implications for intervention development and policy decisions.

Drug Use Initiation and Progression Phase

The initial stage of addiction is initiation, which occurs when a person attempts a substance for the first time. This can happen at any moment in a person's life, but the National Institute on Drug Abuse reports that the majority of persons who develop an addiction do so before the age of 18 and have a substance use problem by the age of 20.

According to Kandel and others' research, the majority of drug usage starts in the early adolescent years, and nearly no one starts using an illicit substance after the age of Twenty-Nine (29). (Chen and Kandel, 1995). While the causal significance of developmental stages is unknown (Morral et al., 2002), studies have shown that adolescents are much less likely to try marijuana if they have not previously tried an alcoholic beverage or cigarettes; similarly, very few try illicit drugs other than marijuana if they have not previously tried marijuana (Brook et al., 1982; Donovan and Jessor, 1983; Kandel, 1975). As previously stated, the majority of these researches are based on samples with only a few serious drug users.

The reasons why a teenager experiments with drugs might be many, but two prevalent causes are curiosity and peer pressure. This latter decision is taken with the goal of better fitting in with that particular set of peers. Another reason why teenagers are more inclined than other age groups to attempt a new substance is that their prefrontal cortex has not yet fully formed. This has an impact on their decision-making process, and many teenagers make decisions without fully contemplating the long-term ramifications of their actions.

However, regardless of starting sequences, age at first use of alcohol, cigarettes, or illicit drugs has been found to be a strong predictor of eventual consequences and dependency. According to epidemiological and clinical studies, teenagers who start taking drugs at a young age use them more frequently, climb to greater levels of use more quickly, and are more likely to keep using them (Anthony and Petronis, 1995; Yu and Williford, 1992).

Just because someone has used a drug does not guarantee that they will become addicted to it. In many circumstances, a person will try a substance out of curiosity and then quit using it after their interest has been fulfilled. Other aspects connected to the drug's function in the individual's life can also influence this decision, such as:

- Drug availability
- Peer use
- Family background and drug history
- Mental health (conditions like depression and anxiety often encourage use)

If the circumstances are favorable and the person continues to use the drug, they may soon enter the second stage of addiction.

Experimentation Phase

The user has progressed beyond simply trying the substance on its own and is now experimenting with it in various settings to see how it affects their life. In general, the medication is associated with social acts during this period, such as experiencing pleasure or unwinding after a long day. It is used by teens to improve party atmospheres or handle stress from homework. Adults explore primarily for the fun of it or to relieve stress.

There are little to no urges for the substance throughout this stage, and the user is still making a conscious decision about whether or not to use it. They may use it impulsively or in a controlled manner, and the frequency with which they do so is largely determined by the person's temperament and rationale for doing so. There is no dependency at this time, and the person can still easily stop using the medicine if they choose to.

Frequent Use Phase

The use of a substance gets normalized as a person continues to experiment with it, and it progresses from occasional to regular use. This does not imply that they utilize it on a daily basis, but rather that there is a pattern to it. The pattern varies according on the person, but some examples include taking it every weekend or during times of mental distress such as loneliness, boredom, or stress. At this moment, social users can start taking their substance on their own, removing the social element from their decision.

At this time, drug usage can become troublesome and have a negative impact on a person's life. After a night of drinking beer or smoking marijuana, the person may begin turning up to work hungover or high. Although there is no addiction at this point, the person is more likely to think about their chosen substance and may have begun to establish a mental reliance on it. When this happens, quitting becomes more difficult, but still achievable without outside assistance.

Risky Use Phase

The distinction between frequent use and dangerous use/abuse is blurry, but it's commonly characterized as continuing to take drugs despite severe social and legal consequences. What started off as a harmless diversion might swiftly escalate into more severe issues. If the medication is not used, the warning signs of addiction will start to appear: yearning, preoccupation with the substance, and symptoms of depression, irritability, and weariness.

The individual's regular use has progressed to the point that it is now having a negative influence on their lives. While a periodic hangover at work or at an event is tolerable in the Frequent Phase, it becomes a regular occurrence in the Risky Phase, and its consequences become evident. Many drinkers are arrested for Driving under the Influence at this time, and everyone's work or school performance will suffer as a result. Frequent use may also result in financial troubles where none previously existed.

People on the outside will almost surely notice a change in the user's conduct at this point, even if the user is unaware of it. The following are some of the most common changes to look for in a drug user:

- Changing peer groups
- Visiting several doctors or rapidly changing doctors
- Hiding medications in easily accessible areas (like mint tins) (if using a prescription drug)
- Losing interest in previous pastimes
- Taking out loans or stealing money
- Ignoring commitments like job or family
- Trying to conceal their drug use

Dependence Phase

Drug dependence develops over time when neurons adjust to only function normally in the presence of the drug. The lack of the substance triggers a variety of physiological effects, ranging from moderate in the instance of coffee to potentially fatal in the case of heroin. Some chronic pain patients are addicted to opioids and need medical help to stop using them.

Drug dependence is described as a psychological and physical state in which a person feels compelled to use a drug on a continuous or periodic basis in order to experience its psychological effects and to avoid the discomfort of its absence.

When a person enters the Dependence Phase, their drug usage is no longer recreational or medical, but rather owing to a dependency on the substance of choice. This is sometimes considered as a broad stage that covers tolerance development and reliance, but the individual should have already established tolerance by this point. As a result, this stage should only be defined by a physical, psychological, or both reliance.

When it comes to physical dependence, the person has overused their chosen drug for long enough that their body has become accustomed to it and has learnt to rely on it. If you quit using something suddenly, your body will go through withdrawal. This is marked by a negative rebound accompanied by unpleasant and occasionally dangerous symptoms that should be addressed by medical personnel. Individuals frequently opt to continue using rather than seek help since it is the simplest and fastest way to avoid withdrawal.

Some substances, particularly prescription pharmaceuticals, can lead to this stage through psychological dependence before a physical dependence develops. When this occurs, the person believes that they must use the substance in order to operate normally. Typically, the medication is used as a coping technique during difficult times, and subsequently it is used in situations where it is not actually essential. A patient using pain medication, for example, may begin to over-medicate because moderate pain is perceived as severe pain.

In each situation, the person takes the substance because they have come to the realization that they require it in some way in order to live. Addiction is almost certain once this thinking takes hold.

Addiction Phase

Drug addiction is a chronic illness marked by obsessive, or uncontrollable, drug seeking and use despite negative effects and long-term brain alterations. Those who abuse medications, whether prescription or illicit, may develop detrimental habits as a result of the alterations.

Drug addiction, also known as substance use disorder, is an illness that affects a person's brain and behavior, causing them to lose control over the use of legal or illegal drugs or medications. Drugs include substances such as alcohol, marijuana, and nicotine. You may continue to use the substance despite the harm it causes if you are addicted (Amaro et'al, 1995).

Though the terms are similar and are commonly associated with drug usage, they are distinct. One of the most significant distinctions is that when someone develops an addiction, drug usage is no longer a conscious choice. It's still a shadow of one until then.

Individuals at this stage believe they can no longer cope with life without their preferred substance, and as a result, they lose total control over their decisions and behaviors.

Addiction danger and speed of addiction differ per substance. Opioid medicines, for example, have a higher risk of addiction and create addiction faster than other drugs.

To become high, you may require more dosages of the substance over time. You may soon require the medicine simply to feel well. You may discover that going without the substance becomes more difficult as your drug use rises. Stopping drug usage can lead to extreme cravings and make you physically unwell (withdrawal symptoms).

The user will likely give up their prior activities and aggressively shun friends and family as a result of the behavioral adjustments that occurred in Stage 4. When questioned about their drug usage, they may feel compelled to lie and become irritated if their way of life is challenged in any way. Users may also be so disconnected from their previous lives at this point that they are oblivious to how their actions are harming them and their relationships.

Addiction is sometimes known as a drug use disorder, which is a fair definition because it is a chronic condition with long-term consequences. Even after quitting a drug and receiving therapy, there is always the possibility of recurrence. This indicates that in order to continue a life of recovery, one must commit to a complete lifestyle transformation.

It might be tough to tell the difference between typical teenage angst and drug usage. The following are some signs that an adolescent or other family member is abusing drugs:

- **School or job problems**, such as frequent absences, a sudden lack of interest in school activities or work, or a reduction in grades or work performance
- **Physical health problems**, such as a lack of energy and ambition, weight gain or loss, or red eyes
- **Neglected appearance** – disinterest in clothes, grooming, or appearance
- **Behavioral changes**, such as exaggerated efforts to keep family members out of his or her room or secrecy about where he or she travels with friends; or significant changes in conduct and relationships with family and friends.
- **Money problems** – unexpected requests for money with no acceptable explanation; or discovering that money is missing or has been stolen, or that objects have vanished from your house, indicating that they may be sold to fund drug use.

Crisis / Treatment Phase

The breaking point in a person's life is the final stage of addiction. Once there, the person's addiction has spiraled out of control, posing a major threat to their health. It's also known as the crisis stage since the addict is most at risk of dying from an overdose or experiencing another traumatic life event at this period.

While a crisis is the worst-case scenario for this period, there is a positive alternative. Many people first seek help from a rehab clinic to begin receiving treatment, either on their own or as a consequence of a crisis. As a result, this stage could signal the end of their addiction and the beginning of a new life free of drugs and alcohol, one that is full of optimism for the future.

It's critical to seek help as soon as possible, regardless of your stage of drug use, especially if you've reached the point where you can't stop using drugs on your own. Addiction is a chronic sickness that only gets worse if left untreated. Addiction is, thankfully, a treatable disorder. Inpatient treatment, outpatient treatment, 12-Step programs, and holistic therapies are among options for drug addiction treatment.

One thing to consider when choosing a drug addiction program is if it offers dual diagnosis treatment. Oftentimes a person will develop a drug addiction after trying to self-medicate symptoms of a mental illness. Other times symptoms of mental illness, such as depression and anxiety, will develop due to chronic drug use. The result is a never-ending cycle that is difficult to break without treating both the drug addiction and the mental illness. Proper assessment of a dual diagnosis can help you in any stage of drug use and addiction.

Summary

Drug misuse is a multifaceted problem that impacts individuals, families, and society as a whole. The physical, psychological, and social levels of individuals and society are all affected as a result of teenage drug addiction. Withdrawal symptoms include psychomotor, palpitation, perspiration, sleeplessness, restlessness, transitory hallucination or illusion, frustration, bodily and psychological ailments, and so on.

Drug misuse, cultivation, and trafficking of illicit narcotics and psychoactive substances are without a doubt a thorn in the flesh in Nigeria and the rest of the world; it is a heinous deed in our society that causes confusion among the majority of our youth. It is a rapidly developing global issue that is currently a public health concern. Drug misuse poses a serious threat to the social, health, and economic fabric of families, societies, and even countries. Almost every country in the world is afflicted by citizens abusing one or more drugs.

REFERENCES:

1. Amaro, H. and Hardy-Fanta, C. (1995). Gender relations in addiction and recovery. Journal of Psychoactive Drugs 27, pp. 325–337.
2. Anglin, M. D., Booth, M. W., Ryan, T. M. and Hser, Y. (1988). Ethnic differences in narcotics addiction. II. Chicano and Anglo Addiction Career Patterns. International Journal of the Addictions 23(10), pp. 1011–1027.
3. Brook, J. S.,Whiteman, M., and Gordon, A. S. (1982). Qualitative and quantitative aspects of adolescent drug use: interplay of personality, family, and peer correlates. Psychological Reports 51(3), pp. 1151– 1163

SECTION TWO:

CANNABINOID ABUSE AND MISUSE: ITS CONNECTED IMPACT ON HEALTH AND WELLBEING

Cannabinoids

Cannabinoids are chemicals found naturally in the Cannabis sativa plant. Only around 66 of the plant's roughly 480 distinct chemicals are classified as cannabinoids.

The term "cannabinoid" refers to any chemical molecule that binds to the body's and brain's cannabinoid receptors and has effects comparable to those generated by the Cannabis Sativa plant, regardless of structure or origin. Recreational, medical, and synthetic cannabinoids are the three forms of cannabinoids that individuals use (Fundacion, 2022).

The cannabis plant generates between 80 and 100 cannabinoids, as well as roughly 300 non-cannabinoid compounds, according to research. THC (delta-9-tetrahydrocannabinol) and CBD (cannabidiol) are the two primary cannabinoids (CBD). The molecule responsible for the psychoactive effects of cannabis, delta-9-tetrahydrocannabinol (THC), is the most well-known of the two.

THC has significant psychoactive effects, meaning it makes a person 'high,' but CBD is considered to have an anti-psychoactive action that reduces or moderates the 'high' induced by THC. CBD is also considered to alleviate some of the other negative effects that THC may cause, such as anxiety.

Another major component is cannabidiol (CBD), which accounts for roughly 40% of the plant resin extract (Hruba et'al, 2014).

Classes of Cannabinoids

The cannabinoids are separated into the following subclasses:

- Cannabigerols (CBG)
- Cannabichromenes (CBC)
- Cannabidiol (CBD)
- Tetrahydrocannabinol (THC)
- Cannabinol (CBN)
- Cannabinodiol (CBDL)
- Other cannabinoids including cannabicyclol (CBL), cannabielsoin (CBE) and cannabitriol (CBT)

The endocannabinoid system

The endocannabinoid system is a complex communication system present in the brain and body that has a wide range of effects. It's made up of cannabinoids, which are natural chemicals, and the channels via which they interact. These components operate together to control a variety of functions, including mood, memory, sleep, and hunger.

What do Cannabinoids do?

Cannabinoids, like opioids, create their effects by interacting with particular receptors found throughout the central nervous system. Simply explained, cannabinoids control how cells communicate, including how they send, receive, and process information.

How are they used?

Cannabinoids, both illicit and synthetic, are often smoked, vaporized, or consumed. Raw (botanical) cannabis, which may be vaporized for therapeutic purposes, as well as oils, liquids, and oral sprays, are all examples of pharmaceutical or medicinal cannabinoids. Gels for direct application to the skin have also been created.

Effects of Cannabinoids

Cannabinoids work by engaging with particular cannabinoid receptors on the surface of cells to produce their effects. CB1 and CB2 are the two primary kinds of cannabinoid receptors in the body, and they are present in various regions of the central nervous system.

Anandamide, a naturally occurring chemical found in the brain that binds to CB1, was identified in 1992. Endocannabinoids are cannabinoid-like chemicals, as well as others that have since been found.

Cannabinoids have different effects depending on which part of the brain is engaged. Memory, cognition, and psychomotor performance may be affected by impacts on the limbic system; reward and pleasure responses may be affected by effects on the mesolimbic pathway; and pain perception may be influenced by effects on the mesolimbic route.

When cannabis is smoked or vaporized, the effects can be felt instantly, or within an hour or two if it is consumed. The following are some of the most common side effects:

- Exhilaration
- Feelings of well-being
- Spontaneous laughter and enthusiasm
- Increased appetite

- Dry mouth
- Calm and introspective mood (Hruba et'al, 2014).

Cannabinoids and other Drugs

Cannabis' interactions with other substances, such as alcohol, prescription pharmaceuticals, and over-the-counter treatments, are frequently unexpected.

When alcohol and cannabis are used together, the negative effects can be amplified, including nausea, vomiting, and feelings of panic, anxiety, and paranoia.

Cannabinoids are used by some people to 'come down' from stimulants like amphetamines and ecstasy. Cannabis and ecstasy use has been related to decreased motivation, memory impairment, and mental health issues.

Health and safety

There is no such thing as a safe amount of drug consumption. Any medicine has a risk associated with it. When using any kind of medication, it's critical to be cautious.

Use of cannabinoids is likely to be more dangerous:

- When cannabis are used in conjunction with alcohol or other drugs, particularly stimulants like crystal methamphetamine ('ice') or ecstasy, they are more harmful.
- When driving or operating heavy machinery, judgment or motor coordination are necessary (in case medical assistance is required)
- When the individual has a mental health issue
- When the individual has a pre-existing cardiac condition

Dependence and tolerance

Regular cannabis usage, especially when begun in youth, is linked to dependency and long-term cognitive impairment (e.g., lower IQ), worse educational outcomes, lower life satisfaction and performance, and a higher risk of psychotic illnesses.

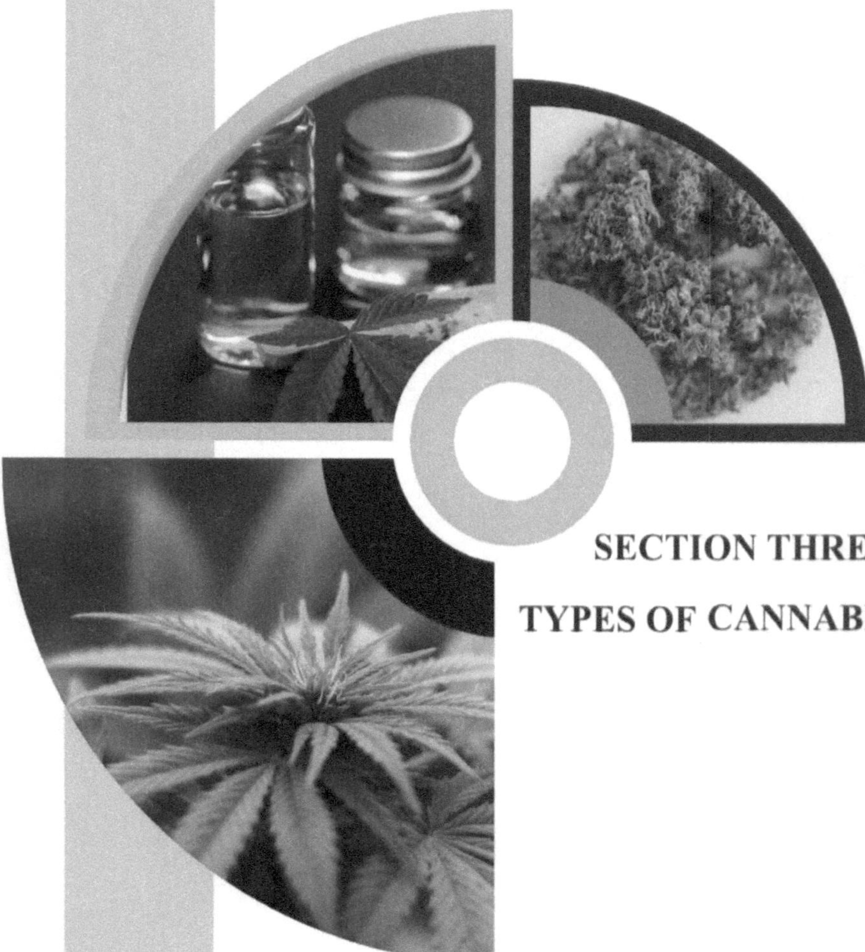

SECTION THREE:

TYPES OF CANNABINOID

UNIT ONE:

BUTANE HASH OIL

The use of concentrated butane hash oil is referred to as dabs or dabbing (or BHO). Inhalation of highly concentrated tetrahydrocannabinol (THC), the main active ingredient in cannabis, is a relatively recent method of administering/ingesting cannabis. Butane oil is used in a chemical procedure to create this concentrated form. To extract the oils from the cannabis, butane is employed.

Chemical Structure of Butane

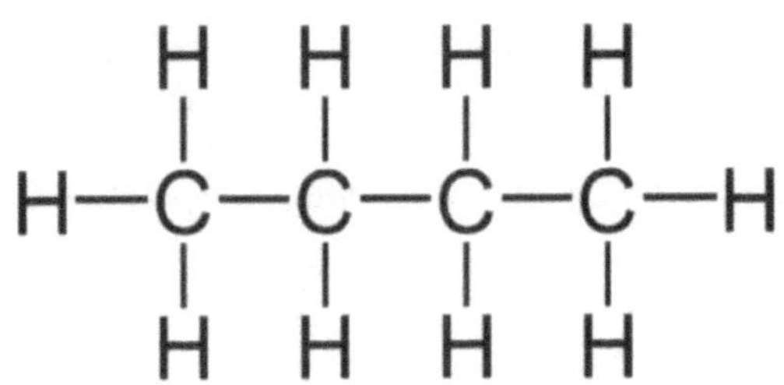

BHO Extraction got its name from Butane, a light hydrocarbon. This extraction method is from the 1970s, and because Butane is so volatile, it can be extremely dangerous if not done correctly. Butane gas flows through the cannabis in a sealed cylinder during the BHO extraction process, separating cannabinoids and terpenes from the raw marijuana plant material (Stogner et'al, 2015) .

Other names

BHO, Marijuana wax, budder, honeycomb, shatter, dab, amber, oil, wax butter, sap

How is it used?

Cannabis is commonly smoked in 'joints,' 'bongs,' or vaporized, however these methods are ineffective for consuming butane hash oil since it turns into a 'runny liquid' when heated. It is typical to employ a specially engineered 'bong,' sometimes known as a 'oil rig.'

Due to the high strength of dabs, which minimizes the number of times it must be consumed to achieve a 'high,' anecdotal research suggests that individuals believe dabbing is a safer way of cannabis intake than a bong or joint.

The home manufacturing of BHO (also known as blasting) has been reported to be dangerous because butane is combustible and very volatile, resulting in a number of mishaps such as explosions, fires, and severe burns.

Nothing is known regarding the risks of 'dabs' when compared to ordinary cannabis, but it has been hypothesized that the increased THC concentration and unique mode of administration may increase the risk of addiction and intensify withdrawal symptoms (Stogner et'al, 2015).

Effects of BHO

There is no such thing as a safe level of drug consumption. Any medicine has a risk associated with it. When using any kind of medication, it's critical to be cautious.

Every person is affected differently by butane hash oil. On different instances or throughout their lives, the same person may have a different experience. Size, weight, and health appear to be some of the factors that influence these differences, whether the person is used to taking it, whether other drugs are taken around the same time, the amount taken, the strength of the drug, expectations of consuming cannabis, the individual's environment and the individual's personality.

Low to moderate cannabis consumption can cause the following side effects:

- Pleasure and relaxation
- Spontaneous laughing and excitement
- Enhanced sociability
- Increased hunger
- Dry mouth

The effects of high-potency cannabis in the form of butane hash oil include:

- Pain relief
- Relaxation
- Nausea reduction
- Changes in heart rate and blood pressure
- Excitement and restlessness
- Confusion and paranoia
- Anxiety and panic
- Lowered attention rate
- Decreased reaction times
- Detachment from reality (Scott et'al, 2018)

Long term effects

The long-term effects of cannabis are influenced by how much and how often it is ingested, as well as how it is consumed (e.g. vaporising a concentrate versus smoking the flower).

- Heavy, frequent cannabis usage can lead to:
- Tolerance to the effects of cannabis
- Reliance on cannabis
- Cognitive impairment

Withdrawal

There is some evidence that the use of higher potency cannabis is linked to a higher risk of cannabis-related issues such as increasing tolerance and withdrawal intensity. Giving up cannabis after a long period of regular, heavy use is difficult since the body must adjust to life without it. Although withdrawal symptoms may only last a week, sleep may be disrupted for much longer. Anxiety, irritability, loss of appetite, and an upset stomach are all possible symptoms, as are sweating, chills, and tremors, as well as disturbed sleep and nightmares (Scott et'al, 2018).

UNIT TWO:

CANNABIDOL

CBD is a molecule found in the Cannabis sativa plant, generally known as hemp or cannabis. The Cannabis sativa plant contains over 80 compounds known as cannabinoids. The most well-known component of cannabis is delta-9-tetrahydrocannabinol (THC). CBD, on the other hand, is derived from hemp, a type of Cannabis sativa plant that has just trace quantities of THC. CBD appears to have impacts on certain brain chemicals, although they are not the same as THC's. Cannabinoids work by interacting with the body's cannabinoid receptors, which are found all over the body and brain and control how a person feels, moves, and reacts.

The second most common active component in cannabis is cannabidiol (marijuana). CBD is obtained straight from the hemp plant, a cousin of marijuana, or created in a lab, and is a key component of Medicinal Marijuana. CBD is one of hundreds of ingredients in marijuana, but it does not produce a "high" on its own. According to a World Health Organization (WHO) report. "CBD has no effects in humans that suggest it could be abused or become addictive.... To date, there has been no indication of any public health issues linked to the usage of pure CBD."

Chemical Structure of Cannabidol

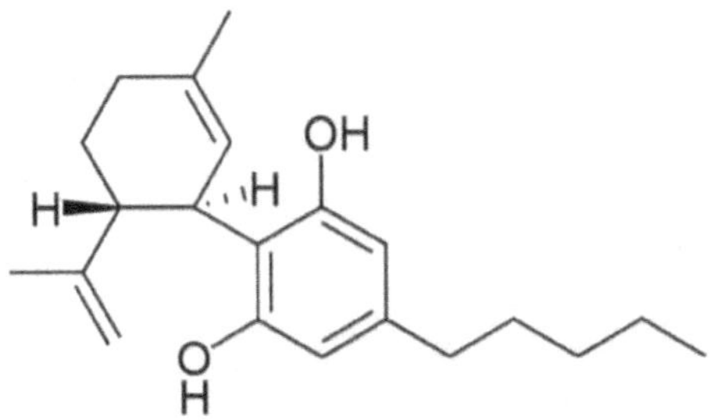

CBD in a prescription form is used to treat epilepsy. CBD is also used to treat anxiety, pain, dystonia, Parkinson's disease, Crohn's disease, and a variety of other ailments, but there is no clear scientific evidence to back up these claims (Boehnke et'al, 2021).

What does it look like?

CBD is normally in the form of oil, but it can also be found in gummies and other sweets. Other options include pills and capsules, creams, lotions, ointments, balms, and vape pens.

Other Names

CBD, diet dabs

How is it used?

CBD can be swallowed, eaten, vapourised and rubbed onto the body.

Effects of CBD

There is no such thing as a safe level of drug consumption. Any medicine has a risk associated with it. When using any kind of medication, it's critical to be cautious.

CBD is possibly safe to use in adequate doses when taken by mouth. Doses as high as 200 mg per day have been successfully administered for up to 13 weeks. A specialized prescription CBD product (Epidiolex) has been used at higher doses and for longer periods of time under the supervision of a healthcare provider.

Dry mouth, low blood pressure, lightheadedness, and sleepiness are all possible adverse effects of CBD. High doses of Epidiolex, a prescription version of CBD, have also been linked to signs of liver harm.

When applied to the skin, there isn't enough trustworthy data to say whether CBD is safe or what the potential adverse effects are.

CBD affects people differently depending on their size, weight, and health; whether they are habituated to taking it; whether they are taking other drugs at the same time; the amount consumed; the strength of the substance (which varies from batch to batch); and the surroundings (where the drug is taken).

CBD does not provide a euphoric or euphoric impact.

Although there is a scarcity of high-quality scientific studies on CBD, we do know that people who use it have claimed relief from a range of ailments, including pain .

The effects of CBD might include:

i. Pain relief: CBD has been shown in studies to help with chronic pain and inflammation. Symptoms of rheumatic disorders, such as fibromyalgia, may also improve with CBD.

ii. Anxiety relief: CBD has been demonstrated to alleviate several symptoms of anxiety disorder.

iii. Relief from cancer treatment side effects: CBD may help to minimize cancer treatment adverse effects such as vomiting and nausea.

iv. Seizures: CBD has been shown to be useful in treating seizures caused by a variety of medical disorders. Epidiolex®, a prescription CBD medicine, has been approved for the treatment of seizures associated with Dravet syndrome, a severe form of epilepsy, by Australia's Pharmaceutical Benefits Scheme (PBS).

v. Possible sleep improvement: CBD may help people with some sleep problems sleep better, but more research is needed (Boehnke et'al, 2021).

Common reported side effects include:

- Diarrhoea
- Tiredness and lethargy
- Dry mouth and
- Loss of appetite are also symptoms.

Long-term effects

Although more research into the long-term effects of CBD is needed, early data suggest that CBD has no long-term harm.

Tolerance and reliance on others

CBD does not appear to have any addictive properties.

Mixing CBD with other drugs

When CBD is combined with other pharmaceuticals, such as over-the-counter or other prescriptions, the results might be unpredictable and harmful.

i. CBD + alcohol or THC: can increase drowsiness and sedation.

ii. CBD + blood thinning medications (Warfin®): can cause higher levels of Warfin® to be present in the body, which may cause excess bleeding and haemorrhage.

UNIT THREE:

CANNABIS

Cannabis is a cannabinoid substance. The amount of various cannabinoids found in the cannabis sativa plant is still being investigated, although it mostly contains the psychoactive cannabinoid THC (delta9 tetrahydrocannabinol) and the non-psychoactive cannabinoid CBD (cannabidiol) (CBD). Marijuana is the most frequent name for it.

Cannabis is the generic word for the psychoactive substance obtained from Cannabis sativa, a plant commonly used to alter consciousness and growing in various parts of the world. Cannabis is also known by a variety of other names, including marijuana, hashish, bhang, ganja, dagga, weed, pot, or reefer, to mention a few (Chan et'al, 2017).

Chemical Structure of Cannabis

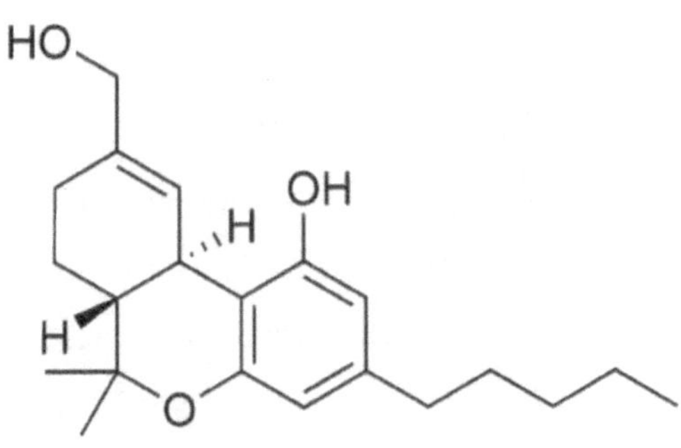

Cannabis has inspired more controversy than any other substance with the potential for abuse. The number of persons who use marijuana is believed to be over 166 million worldwide (UNODC, 2008), and the laws controlling its legal status and potential for medical use vary between and within countries. Many people have questioned its addictive potential. That is, they have questioned whether or not cannabis can lead to dependence or addiction.

The medicinal and psychosocial consequences of cannabis have also been questioned. Some argue that cannabis is dangerous because it serves as a "gateway" drug, leading to the use of more deadly opioids. These factors also make one wonder if effective drugs to aid people in stopping smoking are required.

Other Names

Marijuana, yarndi, pot, weed, hash, dope, gunja, joint, stick, chronic, cone, choof, mull, 420, dabs, dabbing, BHO.

Historical Antecedents of Canabis

Cannabis has a colorful and extensive history. Cannabis was first used in Central Asia or Western China. For millennia, cannabis has been utilized for its purported therapeutic benefits. It was first documented in Emperor Shen Nung's (considered the father of Chinese medicine) pharmacopoeia around 2800 BC. Cannabis has been mentioned in the literature of the Indian Hindus, Assyrians, Greeks, and Romans for medicinal purposes. These writings claimed that cannabis could be used to treat a wide range of ailments, including arthritis, depression, amenorrhea, inflammation, pain, anorexia, and asthma.

According to Hindu mythology, Shiva, the supreme Godhead of various sects, was given the title "Lord of Bhang" because he loved the cannabis plant. The medical advantages of cannabis were considered to be explained by pleasing gods like Shiva, according to ancient Hindus. The start of fever is attributed to the 'hot breath of the gods,' who were enraged by the sick person's behavior, according to ancient Hindu literature. Cannabis was used in religious rites to placate the gods and thereby lower the fever.

According to some sources, cannabis initially appeared in Chinese civilization some four thousand years ago as a plant grown for its fiber, which was used to manufacture clothing, paper, and rope (Abel, 1980). Cannabis has been utilized as a treatment for many diseases and for spiritual rites associated to its mind-altering properties by people from numerous cultures throughout history. For centuries, the value of cannabis as a valuable fiber, its therapeutic potential, and its psychotropic effects and abuse potential have all sparked debate and controversy throughout civilizations.

Based on medical texts outlining its potential medicinal benefits, cannabis was included in the US Pharmacopeia (ca.1870) in the 19th century. Government-sponsored research indicated that cannabis was not "addictive" and had possible health advantages, despite societal anxiety over its usage and repercussions (e.g., Ohio State Medical Society, 1860 and the Indian Hemp Drug Commission, 1895). In the early to mid-1900s, rising cannabis usage in the United States sparked public debate, with some expressing the illogical worry that marijuana use by African Americans and Mexican Americans would lead to marijuana use by white middle and upper class children.

International concerns developed as well, with reports from the International Opium Conference and the League of Nations indicating that certain governments saw the need to regulate cannabis, while others refused. Cannabis was declared a "narcotic" by the International Opium Conference in 1924, and tight controls were imposed. Britain made cannabis illegal in 1941, and the US enacted a Marijuana Transfer Tax and withdrew cannabis from the US Pharmacopeia.

Despite the fact that the New York Academy of Sciences stated in 1944 that public concerns about cannabis were unfounded and that cannabis did not cause addiction, their report detailed a number of negative effects of cannabis use. The National Commission on Marijuana and Drug Abuse in the United States recommended that cannabis possession be decriminalized in 1972. Several US states substituted prison sentences with civil penalties or misdemeanor fines throughout that decade. At the same time, the United States outlawed medicinal cannabis research, while New Mexico approved a bill permitting medical cannabis use.

The Institute of Medicine issued a detailed study in 1999 that acknowledged the possible negative consequences of cannabis, such as addiction, but also made a strong declaration about its medicinal advantages. Legalization and decriminalization debates continue to rage over the world, with no clear consensus in sight and a plethora of national and regional policies as a result.

How is it used?

Cannabis comes in a variety of forms and can be smoked, ingested, or vaporized. The subjective effects of cannabis vary substantially depending on the form taken, according to users.

- Marijuana is the cannabis plant's dried leaves and flowers (buds), which are smoked in a joint or a bong. This is the most typical variant.
- Hashish is a dried plant resin that is commonly blended with tobacco and smoked, as well as added to meals and baked products like cookies and brownies.
- Hash oil is a highly concentrated liquid that is applied to the tip of a joint or cigarette and smoked.

- Concentrates - extracts (dabs, wax, or shatter) made with butane hash oil as a solvent, which are normally vaporized in tiny amounts because to the high THC concentration (Scott et'al, 2018).

Cannabis may be added to a variety of meals known as 'edibles.' It normally takes one to three hours for the effects to become apparent. Impatient or naive users may believe they haven't taken enough to feel the effects, yet consuming more might result in unpleasant powerful psychoactive effects. Even experienced users may find it difficult to limit the amount ingested when edible items have uneven THC levels.

The effects of smoking or vaporizing marijuana are generally noticed right away. Smoking cannabis has been linked to a number of health issues, particularly in the long run. This is especially true when combined with cigarettes.

Cannabis can also be found in synthetic form, which is potentially more hazardous than the actual thing.

Effects of Cannabis

There is no such thing as a safe amount of drug consumption. Any medicine has a risk associated with it. When using any kind of medication, it's critical to be cautious.

Every person is affected differently by cannabis.

Even the same individual might have various experiences on different times or throughout their lives.

Others express anxiety and paranoia, while others claim sensations of relaxation and happiness. Size, weight, and health are some factors that may influence these differences:

- Whether the person is used to taking it
- Whether other drugs are taken around the same time
- The amount taken
- The strength of the drug
- Expectations of consuming cannabis
- The individual's environment
- The individual's personality

The effects of cannabis might include:

- Pleasure and relaxation
- spontaneous laughing and enthusiasm
- enhanced sociability
- increased hunger
- dry mouth

You may also experience:

- memory impairment
- slower reflexes

- bloodshot eyes
- higher heart rate
- moderate anxiety and paranoia if you drink a large amount, powerful batch, or concentrated form.

Long-term Effects

The long-term effects of cannabis are determined by how much, how often, and how it is ingested (e.g. vaporising a concentrate versus smoking the flower).

Its frequent, heavy usage has the potential to cause:

- Tolerance to the effects of cannabis
- Dependency on cannabis
- Cognitive impairment.

Smoking cannabis can also raise your chances of getting a sore throat, asthma, bronchitis, and, if combined with cigarettes, cancer (Stogner et'al, 2015).

Cannabis should not be used by anyone who have a family history of major mental diseases such schizophrenia or bipolar disorder, or who are now experiencing symptoms of these illnesses.

Cannabis usage has been linked to a worsening of bipolar illness, and people who are prone to psychosis (a typical sign of schizophrenia) may be more susceptible to cannabis-induced psychosis. Delusions, hallucinations, and seeing or hearing things that do not exist or are distorted are all signs of psychosis.

Using cannabis with other drugs

The interactions between cannabis and other pharmaceuticals, such as over-the-counter or prescription medications, can be unexpected, and can result in:

- Cannabis + alcohol: nausea, vomiting.
- Cannabis is sometimes used to help with the 'come down' effects
- of stimulant drugs, such as ice, speed and ecstasy.

Withdrawal

Giving off cannabis after a long period of regular, heavy use is difficult since the body must adjust to life without it. Please seek medical advice if you have any concerns (Scott et'al, 2018).

Although withdrawal symptoms may only last a week, sleep may be disrupted for much longer. Anxiety, irritability, lack of appetite, and an upset stomach are among symptoms, as are sweating, chills, and tremors, as well as disturbed sleep and nightmares.

UNIT FOUR:

MEDICINAL CANNABIS

Medicinal cannabis products are high-quality, authorized medications that can be recommended by a physician. Medicinal cannabis is a kind of cannabis that may be used to alleviate the symptoms of certain medical diseases as well as the adverse effects of certain medications.

In general, medicinal cannabis is cannabis that is prescribed to treat the symptoms of a medical disease like epilepsy. It's critical to understand the difference between medical and recreational cannabis. People who want to get 'high' use recreational cannabis (Herbert, 2021).

Chemical Structure of Medicinal Cannabis

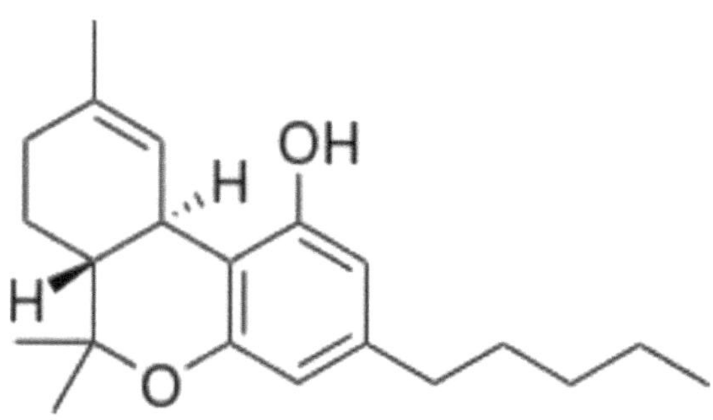

Conventional treatments don't work or don't work as well as medicinal cannabis for some persons with chronic or terminal conditions. Furthermore, traditional drugs may work for certain individuals but have terrible adverse effects that cannabis might assist to alleviate.

There are a variety of medical cannabis medicines available to address various ailments.

Cannabinoids are the active elements in therapeutic cannabis. There are between 80 and 100 different cannabinoids in medicinal cannabis, and scientists are continually learning more about how they all act.

The cannabinoids cannabidiol (CBD) and tetrahydrocannabinol (THC) are present in most therapeutic cannabis products at the time (THC) (Herbert, 2021).

The Endocannabinoid System

The endocannabinoid system is a complex communication system in the brain and body that has a wide range of effects. It's made up of cannabinoids, which are natural chemicals, and the channels via which they interact. These components operate together to control behaviors such as emotion, memory, sleep, and eating. Medicinal cannabis is considered to cure a variety of ailments by working on the endocannabinoid system.

Types and forms of medicinal cannabis

There are three types of cannabis that can be used for medical purposes:

- Pharmaceutical cannabis medications, such as nabiximols (Sativex®) and synthetic cannabinoids like Dronabinol®, that have been approved by the Therapeutic Goods Administration (TGA). Sativex, a nasal or oral spray for treating spasticity caused by multiple sclerosis, has been licensed in over 24 countries.
- Herbal cannabis (plant products) that are controlled and standardized, such as those manufactured in the Netherlands.
- Illegal and unregulated herbal cannabis (plant products), which includes unknown cannabinoid amounts as well as potentially dangerous contaminants like germs and mold (USA only).

Why smoking cannabis for medical purposes is not recommended

Some argue that smoked cannabis should be considered a therapy for a variety of medical ailments, including cancer. However, there are two significant issues to be concerned about.

To begin with, smoking cannabis is a particularly dangerous method of consumption, owing to the direct inhalation of carcinogenic chemicals into the lungs. Health officials advise against smoking cannabis since it has at least 50 of the same carcinogens as cigarettes.

Second, the vast majority of pharmaceuticals are manufactured under stringent guidelines. Doctors who prescribe them (as well as those who use them) will know exactly what's in them this way.

It's critical for doctors to know that drugs have been thoroughly studied and that each dose is same. This implies that doctors can keep track of a drug's effects and modify dosages according on the needs of the patient.

When recreational cannabis is utilized as medication, doctors and patients have no way of knowing how potent it is or what chemical combination it contains. As a result, no two doses will ever be identical (Nazarenus, 2020).

Side effects

Medicines and therapies that can assist lessen the unpleasant symptoms of various illnesses and disorders are in high demand in the society.

Medicinal cannabis in the form of oral extracts, sprays, or tablets has been shown in a growing number of trials to help relieve pain and treat certain conditions. Medicinal cannabis, like many other medications, can have negative side effects such trouble concentrating, dizziness, sleepiness, loss of balance, and cognitive and memory issues.

What medicinal cannabis products are available?

Medicinal cannabis products come in a variety of forms, depending on the symptoms or conditions they're meant to help with. You can also change how you take them. Your doctor will need to analyze your requirements and determine whether a medical cannabis product is right for you.

The bulk of items are imported, however as the Australian medicinal cannabis sector matures, more locally accessible products are expected.

What can medicinal cannabis be used for?

Despite the fact that cannabis, sometimes known as marijuana, has been around for a long time, there is still a lack of official evidence for doctors to use when considering prescription a medical cannabis product to a patient.

Certain medicinal cannabis products may be effective in treating the following illnesses, according to some evidence:

- Epilepsy
- Multiple sclerosis
- Cancer and cancer treatment symptoms (such as nausea, discomfort, and lack of appetite)
- Pain
- Palliative care symptom relief

The Commonwealth Government has produced documents summarizing the evidence to far that medical cannabis may be beneficial in the treatment of certain diseases.

For any medical ailment, a doctor or expert can petition to the government for permission to prescribe medicinal cannabis. The doctor may, however, be required to present evidence that medical cannabis is helpful for the disease being treated. Medical practitioners who prescribe medicinal cannabis can find information and tools from the Office of Medicinal Cannabis (Nazarenus, 2020)..

The Side Effects of Medicinal Cannabis Treatment

Medicinal cannabis drugs, like any prescription medications, might have negative effects. The severity of these effects varies depending on the type of medical cannabis product used and the individual.

In general, CBD-rich products have fewer negative effects than high-THC products, but because CBD dosages in disorders like paediatric epilepsies can be relatively high, a proportion of patients have side effects with these CBD concentrations.

Fatigue and drowsiness, vertigo, nausea and vomiting, fever, reduced or increased appetite, dry mouth, and diarrhoea are all documented adverse effects of medicinal cannabis treatment (both CBD and THC).

Convulsions, feeling euphoric or unsatisfied, sadness, disorientation, hallucinations, paranoid delusions, psychosis, and cognitive distortion have all been linked to THC (and THC-rich drugs) (having thoughts that are not true).

General Cautions

Patients who are using medical cannabis should not drive or operate machines. Furthermore, several days after the last dose, detectable THC (tetrahydrocannabinol - the major psychoactive ingredient in cannabis) concentrations can be discovered in urine. 80 to 90 percent of the dosage may take up to five days to be eliminated. Drunk driving is a criminal offense, and patients should talk to their doctor about the consequences for safe and legal driving.

Medicinal cannabis is not appropriate for:

- Women who are pregnant, wanting to become pregnant, or breastfeeding persons with unstable cardiovascular disease
- Patients with neurological disorders may be more susceptible to the harmful effects of medical cannabis.
- Persons who have a psychosis or mood or anxiety condition that is active or has been active in the past
- Persons having a heart condition that is in a state of flux

For many illnesses and symptoms, there is no information on the most effective or safe dosage. As a result, initial dosages should be minimal and gradually raised until patients respond positively or the perceived advantages exceed the unfavorable side effects. Low starting dosages are especially crucial for those who have memory and cognitive problems, liver and kidney disease, and bodily weakness and wasting caused by severe chronic illness. Young individuals and the elderly benefit from low starting dosages.

Doctors should:

- Frequently evaluate interactions between medical cannabis and other medications
- Carefully examine elderly and particularly sensitive patients When determining whether to continue or discontinue therapy,
- Consider your liver function.

Especially though there is some proof that medicinal cannabis treatment is beneficial for one ailment or symptom, this does not indicate it will be beneficial for other conditions, even if the product and dose are the same.

There is very little research on how medical cannabis interacts with other drugs that have been licensed (Therapeutic Goods Administration, 2018).

UNIT FIVE:

SYNTHETIC CANNABINOIDS?

Synthetic cannabinoids (also known as synthetic cannabis) are a type of novel psychoactive drug (NPS) that was created to mimic or generate effects comparable to cannabis. It has been available for purchase online since 2004.

Synthetic cannabinoids, on the other hand, are not a synthetic form of cannabis and do not duplicate the effects of THC (delta-9 tetrahydrocannabinol, the active element in cannabis) — instead, they generate a range of undesirable side effects that are not caused by cannabis.

As a result, the labels "synthetic cannabis" and "synthetic marijuana" are misleading (Darke et'al, 2021).

Chemical Structure of Synthetic Cannabinoid

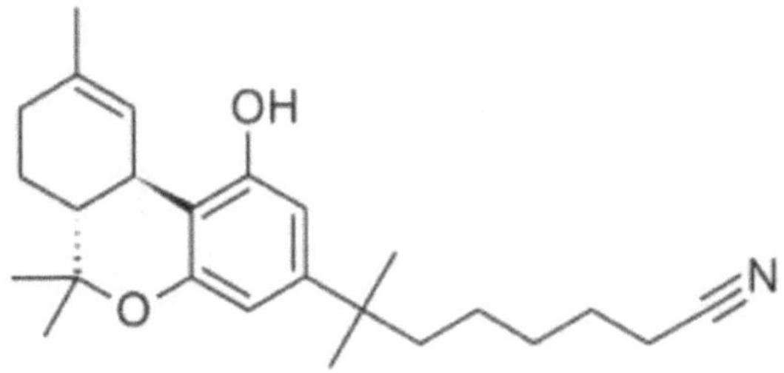

Synthetic cannabinoid receptor agonists (SCRAs) is the actual word for these compounds, however for the sake of convenience, this book shall refer to them as synthetic cannabinoids.

A variety of synthetic cannabis drugs have been developed throughout the years. They are comparable to those found in natural cannabis, but they are more powerful and have been linked to a variety of side effects.

Synthetic cannabinoids are compounds that imitate THC's effects. These synthetic cannabinoids, like THC, target the brain's cannabinoid type 1 receptor (CB1R), which is responsible for THC's euphoric effects (Bright, 2013).

Many of these compounds have evolved to the point that they no longer fit within the cannabinoid categorization system.

What do synthetic cannabinoids look like?

Synthetic cannabinoids are powdered compounds that are mixed with solvents and sprayed on plants before being sold in colorful, branded packets. Because makers try to stay ahead of the law by altering the ingredients in each batch, even if the name and logo on the pack appear to be the same, different packets might have different outcomes.

Other Names

Synthetic cannabinoids are sold under a variety of trade names.

Spice was the first in a line of synthetic cannabis drugs that were offered in a number of European nations. Kronic, Northern Lights, K2, and Kaos are just a few of the comparable items that have been invented since then.

Aphrodisiac tea, herbal incense, and potpourri are all examples of synthetic cannabis.

How are synthetic cannabinoids used?

Smoking synthetic cannabis is the most prevalent method. In most cases, the results are felt within minutes.

Effects of synthetic cannabinoids

There is no such thing as a safe amount of drug consumption. Any medicine has a risk associated with it. When using any kind of medication, it's critical to be cautious.

Synthetic cannabinoids impact people differently depending on their size, weight, and health; if they are habituated to taking it; whether they are taking other drugs at the same time; the amount consumed; the drug's potency (which varies from batch to batch); and the atmosphere (where the drug is taken).

The effects of synthetic cannabinoids can include:

- Exhilaration
- Disorientation

- Lack of coordination
- Rapid and irregular pulse
- Racing thoughts
- Agitation, anxiety, and paranoia
- Psychosis
- Violent and aggressive behavior
- Chest discomfort
- Vomiting
- High blood pressure (hypertension)
- Difficulty breathing
- Hyperthermia (overheating)
- Rhabdomyolysis (muscle tissue breakdown)
- Acute renal damage
- Seizures
- Stroke
- Death

Set and Setting

Synthetic cannabinoids have different affects based on a person's mood (commonly referred to as the 'set') or the environment they are in (often referred to as the 'setting'):

- **Set:** a person's mental state, prior experiences with psychoactive substances, and expectations of what would happen. Before taking synthetic cannabis, for example, emotions of tension or anxiety might be amplified, resulting in an unpleasant experience.

- **Setting:** the atmosphere in which someone consumes synthetic cannabinoids, including whether it's familiar and comfortable, who they're with, whether they're indoors or outside, and the sort of music and light. For example, while utilizing synthetic cannabinoids in a peaceful, quiet, and relaxed atmosphere might be enjoyable, doing it in a noisy, packed one can be unpleasant (Darke et'al, 2021).

Overdose

You might overdose if you take a huge amount or have a very potent batch. If you experience any of the following symptoms, call an ambulance:

- Rapid/irregular heart rate
- Chest discomfort
- Difficulty breathing
- Severe hyperthermia (very high body temperature)
- Delusional behavior

Long-term Effects

Synthetic cannabinoids usage on a regular basis can lead to mental health issues, cardiac difficulties, and behavioural and cognitive impairments. Mental health and synthetic cannabis

Synthetic cannabinoids should be avoided by anyone with mental health problems or a family history of mental health problems.

People who use synthetic cannabinoids are more likely to have anxiety and depression symptoms, and long-term usage has been related to major mental health problems.

After taking synthetic cannabis, even healthy and susceptible people can develop psychosis. Synthetic cannabinoids' psychotic effects are more severe than those associated with cannabis, and they can linger for weeks after last use.

Tolerance and Dependence

People who use synthetic cannabinoids on a daily basis might soon get addicted to them. They may believe they require synthetic cannabinoids to carry out daily tasks such as working, learning, and socializing, or simply to get by. They may also acquire a resistance to it, requiring higher doses of synthetic cannabinoids to get the same effect.

Mixing synthetic cannabinoids with other drugs

When synthetic cannabinoids are combined with other medicines, such as over-the-counter or prescription prescriptions, the results can be unexpected and harmful.

- **Antidepressants + synthetic cannabinoids**: combining antidepressants like SSRIs (selective serotonin reuptake inhibitors) can cause fever, rapid heartbeat, convulsions, organ failure, coma, and death.

- Synthetic cannabinoids combined with stimulants such as ice or cocaine: the effects can be very harmful and increase the probability of experiencing anxiety (Bright, 2013).

NB: ***Use of more than one drug or type of drug consumed at the same time is called polydrug use.***

Withdrawal

Giving off synthetic cannabis after a lengthy period of use is difficult since the body must adjust to life without them.

When persons who use synthetic cannabinoids severely on a regular basis try to quit, they may have withdrawal symptoms such as:

- Sleeplessness
- Nausea and vomiting
- Lack of appetite
- Paranoia
- Panic attacks
- Agitation and irritability
- Anxiety
- Mood swings
- Fast pulse.

By taking regular breaks from smoking the drug and avoiding using a big quantity at once, the danger of tolerance and reliance on synthetic cannabinoids, as well as their side effects, may be decreased.

Health and Safety

Synthetic cannabinoids cannot be used safely. If you do decide to use the medicine, keep the following points in mind:

Regulating intake

- Because the potency of synthetic cannabinoids fluctuates from batch to batch, it's impossible to forecast their intensity and effects (even if they've been used before).
- Starting with a very tiny dose will help you judge the potency and potential side effects.

Taking synthetic cannabinoids without a 'mixer,' such as tobacco or dried parsley, should be avoided at all costs. Inhaling the substance through bongs or pipes, on the other hand, might raise the chance of an overdose or a severe response (Darke et'al, 2021).

Packaging that gives the wrong impression

- Synthetic cannabis' packaging might be deceiving. Despite the fact that the components are adverti

- sed as "herbal," the psychoactive substance is synthetic.It's possible that not all substances or their precise quantities are reported, increasing the danger of overdosing.
- Chemicals vary from batch to batch, thus even though the packaging is same, various packets might have varied effects.

When it should be avoided at all costs

When using synthetic cannabis, you're more prone to Danger if :

- Used with alcohol or other substances, especially stimulants like crystal methamphetamine ('ice') or MDMA
- The person has a mental health condition
- The person has an existing cardiac disease
- The person is driving or operating heavy machinery
- Judgment or motor coordination is required
- The person is alone (in case medical aid is necessary)

Summary

The terms "cannabis" and "marijuana" are frequently used interchangeably, however they do not signify the same substance. All items generated from the Cannabis sativa plant are referred to as "cannabis." Approximately 540 chemical compounds are found in the cannabis plant. Parts of or products from the Cannabis sativa plant that contain significant levels of tetrahydrocannabinol are referred to as "marijuana" (THC).

THC is the active ingredient in marijuana that has the most impact on a person's mental state. THC is present in only a small percentage of cannabis plants. These plants are classified as "industrial hemp" rather than marijuana under US law. The plant Cannabis sativa is referred to as "cannabis" throughout the rest of this data page.

Cannabinoids contain a wide range of medical characteristics, allowing cannabis to be used to treat a variety of ailments (also known as marijuana). Cannabinoids are used in cancer therapy to reduce nausea and stimulate appetite in palliative care, but further in-depth research has revealed that they are also involved in cell division, autophagy, and apoptosis, resulting in the cannabinoid system, a therapeutic and tumor-prevention target.

REFERENCES

1. Stogner J., Miller B. Assessing the Danger of "Dabbing": Mere Marijuana or Harmful New Trend? Pediatrics. 2015;136(1).
2. Colizzi M, Bhattacharyya, S. Cannabis use and the development of tolerance: a systematic review of human evidence. Neuroscience & Biobehavioural Reviews. 2018;93.
3. Scott J, Slomiak, ST., Jones, JD., Rosen, AFG., Moore, TM., Gur, RC. . Association of Cannabis with Cognitive Functioning in Adolescents and Young Adults. . JAMA Psychiatry. 2018;75(6):585-95.
4. Boehnke K GJ, Matallana L, Williams D,. Cannabidiol Use for Fibromyalgia: Prevalence of Use and Perceptions of Effectiveness in a Large Online Survey. The Journal of Pain 2021;22(5).
5. Chan GCK, Hall W, Freeman TP, Ferris J, Kelly AB, Winstock A. User characteristics and effect profile of Butane Hash Oil: An extremely high-potency cannabis concentrate. Drug and Alcohol Dependence. 2017;178:32-8.
6. Darke S, Banister S, Farrell M, Duflou J, Lappin J. 'Synthetic cannabis': A dangerous misnomer. International Journal of Drug Policy [Internet]. 2021 [20.10.2021]; 98:[103396 p.].
7. Nazarenus C. Medical cannabis handbook for healthcare professionals. New York: Springer Publishing Company 2020.
8. Fundacion Canna. What are cannabinoids? Where can cannabinoids be found? n.d. [cited: 03.02.2022].

9. MacCallum CA, Russo EB. Practical considerations in medical cannabis administration and dosing. European Journal of Internal Medicine. 2018;49:12-9.
10. Scott JC, Slomiak ST, Jones JD, Rosen AFG, Moore TM, Gur RC. Association of Cannabis With Cognitive Functioning in Adolescents and Young Adults: A Systematic Review and Meta-analysis. JAMA Psychiatry. 2018;75(6):585-95.
11. Herbert A Hardy J. Medicinal cannabis use in palliative care. Australian Journal of General Practice. 2021;50(6).
12. American Psychiatric Association. Diagnostic and statistical manual of mental disorders. 5th ed. Arlington: American Psychiatric Association; 2013.
13. Hruba L McMahon L. The cannabinoid agonist HU-210: pseudo-irreversible discriminative stimulus effects in rhesus monkeys. European Journal of Pharmacology. 2014 727.
14. Belackova V, Ritter A, Shanahan M, Chalmers J, Hughes C, Barratt M & Lancaster K. (2015). Medicinal cannabis in Australia: framing the regulatory options.
15. Therapeutic Goods Administration. (2018). Guidance for the use of medicinal cannabis in Australia: Patient information: The side effects of medicinal cannabis treatment
16. Bright S. Not for human consumption: new and emerging drugs in Australia. What do clinicians, allied health and youth workers, researchers and policy makers need to know? Melbourne: Alcohol and Drug Foundation; 2013.